YOUR KNOWLEDGE HAS VALUE

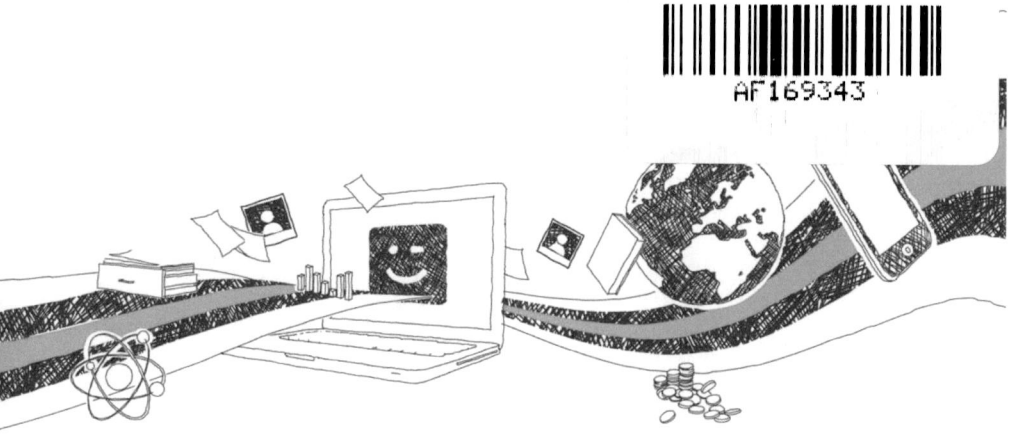

- We will publish your bachelor's and master's thesis, essays and papers

- Your own eBook and book - sold worldwide in all relevant shops

- Earn money with each sale

Upload your text at www.GRIN.com and publish for free

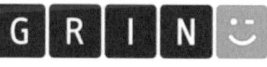

Bibliographic information published by the German National Library:

The German National Library lists this publication in the National Bibliography; detailed bibliographic data are available on the Internet at http://dnb.dnb.de .

This book is copyright material and must not be copied, reproduced, transferred, distributed, leased, licensed or publicly performed or used in any way except as specifically permitted in writing by the publishers, as allowed under the terms and conditions under which it was purchased or as strictly permitted by applicable copyright law. Any unauthorized distribution or use of this text may be a direct infringement of the author s and publisher s rights and those responsible may be liable in law accordingly.

Imprint:

Copyright © 2018 GRIN Verlag
Print and binding: Books on Demand GmbH, Norderstedt Germany
ISBN: 9783668637245

This book at GRIN:

https://www.grin.com/document/411954

Patrick Kimuyu

Drug Nutrient Interactions. The Case for Warfarin's Interaction with Vitamin E and Fish Oil

GRIN Verlag

GRIN - Your knowledge has value

Since its foundation in 1998, GRIN has specialized in publishing academic texts by students, college teachers and other academics as e-book and printed book. The website www.grin.com is an ideal platform for presenting term papers, final papers, scientific essays, dissertations and specialist books.

Visit us on the internet:

http://www.grin.com/

http://www.facebook.com/grincom

http://www.twitter.com/grin_com

Content

Introduction 2

Warfarin and Its Therapeutic Mechanisms 3

Types of Nutrient Drug Interactions Associated with Warfarin 5

Warfarin Interaction with Vitamin E 7

Warfarin Interaction with Fish Oil 8

Conclusion 10

References 11

Introduction

In practice, nutritional components are known to influence the efficacy of therapeutic agents. Some nutrients improve the efficacy of some drugs, whereas others reduce their therapeutic potency. As such, it is critical to understand the nutritional interactions between drugs and the nutritional components in the diet. Diets which interfere with the activity of certain drugs should be avoided during the treatment period. This prevents nutritional interactions which may result into adverse reactions. The same precaution applies to nutritional supplements. Over the past few decades, nutritional supplements have flooded the market. However, these supplements raise safety concerns, especially on dosage, efficacy and side effects. Despite the safety concerns, it is worth noting that some nutritional components such as vitamins and fatty acids have been found to have clinical significance. They are used for the treatment of different health conditions and illnesses, especially when combined with therapeutic agents. For instance, vitamin E and Omega-3 fatty acids have gained immense acceptance in clinical practice. However, their use should be guided by their interactions with drugs. Warfarin, an antithrombotic agent, is one of the drugs which exhibit interactions with vitamin E and fish oil. This drug is used for the prevention and treatment of arterial and venous thrombotic disease since its development. However, dietary interactions have always complicated its safe use (Murphy 2011, p. 351). Therefore, this paper will provide a comprehensive assessment of warfarin and its nutritional interactions, primarily vitamin E and fish oil.

Warfarin and Its Therapeutic Mechanisms

Biologically, the antithrombotic effect of warfarin depends on the drug's pharmacodynamics and pharmacokinetics factors. This implies that an extensive understanding of these factors plays a key role in improving the effectiveness and safety of warfarin therapy (Murphy 2011, p. 351). In addition, it is worth noting that the pharmacokinetics and pharmacodynamics of warfarin differ between the R and S enantiomers. Studies indicate that S-warfarin exhibits more potency than R-warfarin (Paterson et al. 2006). This aspect is attributable to their biological properties, primarily receptor affinity to the key enzymes involved in the synthesis of vitamin K-dependent clotting factors (Murphy 2011, p. 353).

Overall, warfarin is readily absorbable with a 100% bioavailability after an oral administration. Studies indicate that similar pharmacokinetic features are experienced for both intravenous and oral formulations. Following administration, warfarin reaches the peak plasma concentration within 0.3 to 4 hours. However, it is worth noting that the rate of absorption is decreased by food interaction, but this does not influence the extent of the drug's absorption (Murphy 2011, p. 353). Regarding the distribution of warfarin, the volume of distribution is similar to that of albumin with an average volume of 0.15 L/kg. However, warfarin's distribution depends on its protein binding capacity. Studies indicate that more than 98% of warfarin binds to plasma proteins. As a result, only a small percentage of the drug remains free. This implies that the unbound concentration is available for pharmacological activity. Therefore, the concentration of the free warfarin in the plasma increases as plasma albumin concentrations decrease, leading to an increased plasma clearance. On the other hand, the metabolism of warfarin exhibits stereoselectivity. Its elimination occurs almost entirely through metabolism in which hepatic cytochrome P-450 microsomal enzymes catalyze the inactivation of warfarin metabolites. In turn, the hydroxylated metabolites are reduced into warfarin alcohols (hydroxyl warfarins) by reductases. These alcohol derivatives and inactive oxidative residues are eliminated through urinary excretion.

Overall, warfarin is known to exert its thrombotic effect through interfering with blood clotting process. It interferes with the synthesis of the key clotting factors, primarily those whose synthesis depends on the availability of vitamin K. For instance, clotting factors II, VII and IX are synthesized in the hepatic system under the influence of vitamin K. The hepatic synthesis of clotting factor X is also vitamin K-dependent. Biologically, warfarin reduces the levels of vitamin K-dependent clotting factors through inhibiting the activity of the core enzymes, vitamin K1 reductase and vitamin K epoxide reductase (VKOR), which are involved in the synthesis. These enzymes play integral roles in the formation of active clotting factors from their precursor proteins. The mechanism involves gamma-carboxylation of the glutamic acid residues of the clotting factors precursor molecules, primarily at the NH2-terminal to form biologically active clotting factors. During the process of gamma-carboxylation, a reduced form of vitamin K (vitamin KH2) becomes oxidized to form an inactive form, vitamin KO. In order to recycle, VKOR and vitamin K1 reductase convert vitamin KO into vitamin KH2 required for the synthesis of clotting factors. Therefore, warfarin interferes with this hepatic recycling process of vitamin K resulting to low supply of biologically active vitamin K (Ansell et al. 2008). In turn, the inadequate supply of vitamin K leads to a significant decrease in vitamin K-dependent clotting factors, thus preventing blood clotting in the arteries and veins. However, it is worth noting that the biologic effects of warfarin are experienced after the depletion all the previously activated clotting factors in accordance to their half-lives. This is why it takes at least 3 days for its effects to occur after the initiation of therapy.

Another mechanism through which warfarin exerts its antithrombotic effect is the interference with the synthesis of anticoagulant proteins. Clinical studies indicate that warfarin causes interference with the biosynthesis of proteins S and C.

Types of Nutrient Drug Interactions Associated with Warfarin

In understanding the aspect of nutritional interaction of warfarin, it is worth defining the types of drug interactions associated with warfarin. Ordinarily, there are two types of drug interactions, categorized as either pharmacodynamics or pharmacokinetic interactions. Pharmacodynamics interactions are known to enhance or counteract the pharmacologic effect in the body. In the case of warfarin, these interactions result into changes in platelet function or homeostasis. On the other hand, pharmacokinetic interactions alter the drug's absorption and its distribution in the body. They also alter its metabolism, as well as elimination, thus the drug's pharmacological activity is influenced, significantly. Therefore, pharmacokinetic interactions cause changes in serum warfarin concentration. In this context, the interaction between warfarin and nutrients, primarily vitamin E and Fish oil are pharmacodynamics interactions. For instance, vitamin E is known to potentiate the risk of bleeding among patients who are on warfarin therapy (Liu & Stumpo 2007).

From a clinical perspective, the modes of action of warfarin, vitamin E and fish oil exhibit significant differences and similarities. Therefore, these aspects influence the interaction between warfarin and the two nutrients. This implies that understanding warfarin's nutrients interaction requires a brief comparison on their respective modes of action. One of the main similarities among warfarin, vitamin E and fish oil, primarily omega-3 fatty acids is that they are heart protective. As such, they are useful for the prevention, treatment and the management of cardiovascular disease in humans.

As discussed earlier, warfarin exerts its pharmacologic effect by inhibiting the synthesis of anticoagulant proteins and vitamin K-dependent clotting factors. Therefore, the antithrombotic effect of warfarin accounts for its heart protective capacity.

On the other hand, vitamin E exerts its heart protective effect through inhibiting oxidative reactions on cell membranes. Biologically, vitamin E contains α-Tocopherol, a lipid-soluble antioxidant which plays critical antioxidative functions through the glutathione peroxidase pathway. In atherosclerosis, vitamin E prevents the oxidation of LDL cholesterol which contains oxidative –sensitive fatty acids, thus preventing plaque formation in blood vessels. Therefore, it is believed that adequate concentration of vitamin E stabilizes formed plaques in cardiovascular disease and prevents the development of atherosclerosis (Simon et al. 2001). This implies that vitamin E plays some biological roles in the synthesis of vitamin K-dependent clotting factors which is inhibited by warfarin. As such, vitamin E potentiates the effects of warfarin.

Fish oil contains biologically active fatty acids, primarily the omega 3 and omega 6 fatty acids (Calder 2012, p. 1S). Over the decades, fish oil has gained acceptance for medical purposes. The acceptance of fish oil is attributable to its potential health benefits. Some of the physiological roles of fish oil-derived long-chain fatty acids include the regulation of blood pressure, platelet function, blood coagulation, plasma TG concentrations, heart rate, and cardiac function. Therefore, adequate concentrations of fish oil decreases blood pressure and the likelihood of thrombosis. They also increase vascular reactivity and heart rate variability. As such, fish oil helps in the prevention of hypertension, thrombosis, cardiovascular disease, and hypertriglyceridemia (Calder 2012, p. 3S). Contrary to the mechanism of warfarin, long-chain fatty acids in fish oil exhibit a multifactorial mechanism of action. Overall, fish oil-derived omega-3 fatty acids exert their physiological effects in four general mechanisms. First, they influence hormone or metabolite concentration. Through this mechanism, they can influence tissue or cell behaviour. Second, the fatty acids cause direct effects on cell behaviour through fatty acid receptors (Oh et al. 2010). Third, omega-3 fatty acids act by influencing other factors such as oxidative stress and oxidation of LDL. Changes in these factors lead to influences on cell and tissue behaviour. Finally, these fatty acids cause their physiological effects through changes in cell membrane phospholipids-mediated cell behaviour (Calder 2012, p. 3S). In comparison to warfarin, especially based on the antithrombotic effect, fish oil decreases platelet function and blood coagulation the same roles played by warfarin but their mechanisms of action are different. In general, fish oil potentiates the effects of warfarin.

Warfarin Interaction with Vitamin E

Over the past decade, dietary interaction between warfarin and vitamin E has been under intensive scientific inquiry. This inquiry was caused by preliminary reports that generated contradictory evidence on the potential interaction between warfarin and dietary supplements, primarily vitamin E (Kim & White 1996). One of the initial studies on vitamin E interaction with warfarin was conducted by Corrigan and his colleagues in 1974. This study investigated the effect of hypervitaminosis E in humans. Earlier studies on animals showed that excess intakes of vitamin E were associated with haemorrhagic state and prolonged prothrombin time. This phenomenon had not been reported in normal humans. However, this study was the first to document possible interactions between vitamin E and warfarin. According to the results of this study, a patient who was taking vitamin E while on warfarin and clofibrate therapy developed acchymoses accompanied by prolonged prothrombin time. In contrast, the discontinuation of vitamin E ingestion led to a reversal of prothrombin time to baseline levels. Another significant finding recorded in this study was the decrease of vitamin K-dependent clotting factors. However, platelet function remained at normal levels (Corrigan Jr. & Marcus 1974). Another significant study, which was done in 2000 to determine potential interaction between warfarin and alternative therapies, showed vitamin E as a potential anticoagulant. This study was based on documented reports of products with potential interaction with warfarin. However, the study suggested for further studies to confirm the clinical significance of the interaction (Heck, DeWitt & Lukes 2000). Tjhis study was followed by a similar investigation in 2001 that provided theoretical evidence of vitamin E interaction with warfarin. In this study, it was concluded that a concomitant use of vitamin E with warfarin generated antiplatelet effect, as well as increasing the anticoagulant effect of warfarin (Stenton, Bungard & Ackman 2001).

Consequently, recent studies on this issue have produced clinical evidence that shows vitamin E has potential interactions with warfarin. One of the most convincing evidence on the effects of vitamin E on the International Normalized Ratio (INR) is the increase of anticoagulation. It is apparent that vitamin E decreases the concentration of clotting components in blood. As such, it potentiates the effects of blood thinners including warfarin. According to the current clinical studies, vitamin E has been found to exert blood-thinning effects. This implies that individuals who are on blood-thinning medications should observe caution when taking vitamin E supplements. These studies suggest that intake of up to 800 IU among individuals on warfarin therapy is relatively safe. On the other hand, vitamin E doses above 1, 000 IU have been found to increase the risk of bleeding.

Warfarin Interaction with Fish Oil

Fish oil has also been suggested to cause a potential interaction with warfarin. Over the past decade, several studies have been carried out to determine the effect of fish oil in patients undergoing warfarin therapy. However, initial studies did not generate conclusive evidence on any possible interaction. For instance, a clinical study by Norwegian researchers investigated the long-term effects of fish oil on bleeding episodes and homeostatic variables among heart disease patients who were on aspirin or warfarin therapy. In this study, 511 patients were selected to participate in the study. These patients were put on fish oil containing eicosapentaenoic acid (EPA), docosahexanoenoic acid (DEA) and vitamin E in the ratio of 2 g, 1.3 g and 14.8 mg, daily. They were then randomized to receive 4g of fish oil and 300 mg of warfarin per day. This was followed by 3-months evaluation intervals for 9 months. According to the results of this study, fish oil supplementation did not show statistically significant bleeding risks in the patients. However, some clinical changes were observed. For instance, a 19.1% decrease in serum triglyceride levels was noted. In addition, fish oil was found to increase episodes of gastrointestinal bleeding and nosebleeds. Overall, there was a significant increase of serum phospholipid levels of EPA AND DEA among the patients. Despite these clinical implications, it was concluded that fish oil did not produce significant long-term effects on fibrinolysis and coagulation in patients taking warfarin (Eritsland et al. 1995).

In another study which was carried out at the University of Texas Health Science centre, fish oil supplementation did not show significant interaction with warfarin. In this study, researchers aimed at determining the effects of fish oil supplementation on INR among patients on warfarin therapy. This was a placebo-controlled, double-blind, randomized study involving 11 participants who had deep vein thrombosis, prosthetic heart valves, or cardiomyopathy with stable INR values which had been achieved within 4 weeks of warfarin therapy. These participants received a placebo of 3-6 grams per day of fish oil for 4 weeks. INR values were then measured twice weekly over the entire trial period. According to the results of this study, there were no significant changes in INR values among the patients. This implied that fish oil supplementation with up to 6 grams per day did not result into significant interactions with warfarin, primarily on bleeding incidence and INR changes (Bender et al. 1998).

Despite these revelations, a recent study carried out by researchers at Shawnee Mission Medical Centre, Kansas show evidence of clinically significant interaction between fish oil and warfarin.

This research involved a 67-year-old woman who had experienced numerous health problems including coronary artery disease, hyperlipidemia, hypothyroidism, heart attack, and osteopenia. She was taking warfarin in combination with other drugs including conjugated oestrogens, bisoprolol, aspirin, lisinopril, atorvastatin, and levothyroxine. She was also supplementing with 1 gram a day of fish oil and 400UI of vitamin E, daily. Initially, this woman had achieved a stable NRI between 2 to 3 in 5 months, while on a warfarin therapy of 1.5 mg per day. When she doubled her daily fish oil dosage, in March 2002, her INR value rose from 2.8 to 4.1 within a month. This was followed by a drop of NRI value from 4.1 to 1.6 after she returned to her initial dosage of 1 gram of fish oil per day. In conclusion, researchers in this study suggested that the high dose of fish oil might have been responsible for the additional anticoagulation effect indicated by a higher INR. However, it was also concluded that 1 gram a day of fish oil did not show significant effects on NRI (Buckley, Goff & Knapp 2004).

Conclusion

Conclusively, it is apparent that there are potential interactions between warfarin and the two dietary components; vitamin E and fish oil. According to the recent studies, excessive intake of vitamin E while on warfarin therapy increases the risk of bleeding. On the other hand, it is evident that fish oil affects platelet aggregation. It is also believed to affect the functions of vitamin K-dependent clotting factors. One of the most possible ways through which fish oil can affect the function of platelets is through decreasing thromboxane A (2) concentrations within platelets. Despite the insufficiency of the existing research on warfarin and dietary interactions, primarily with vitamin E and fish oil, high doses of these supplements seem to be associated with adverse effects.

References

Ansell, J, Hirsh, J, Hylek, E, Jacobson, A & Crowther, M 2008, 'The pharmacology and management of the vitamin K antagonists. American College of Chest Physicians Evidence-Based Clinical Practice Guidelines (8th edition)', *Chest*, vol. 133 no 6, pp. 160s-98s.

Bender, NK, Kraynak, MA & Chiquette, E 1998, 'Effects of marine fish oils on the anticoagulation status of patients receiving chronic warfarin therapy', *Journal of Thrombosis and Thrombolysis*, vol. 5, pp. 257-61.

Calder, P 2012, Mechanisms of action of (n-3) fatty acids', *The Journal of Nutrition*, viewed 27 November 2017, < http://jn.nutrition.org/content/early/2012/01/24/jn.111.155259.full.pdf >

Corrigan Jr., JJ & Marcus, F 1974, 'Coagulopathy associated with vitamin E ingestion', *JAMA*, vol. 230 no. 9, pp. 1300-1301.

Eritsland, J., et al. 1995, 'Long-term effects of n-3 polyunsaturated fatty acids on haemostatic variables and bleeding episodes in patients with coronary artery disease', *Blood Coagulation and Fibrinolysis*, vol. 6, pp. 17-22.

Heck, AM, DeWitt, BA & Lukes, A 2000, 'Potential interactions between alternative therapies and warfarin', *American Journal of Health-System Pharmacy*, vol. 57 no. 13, pp. 1221-1227.

Kim, JM &White, RH, 'Effect of vitamin E on the anticoagulant response to warfarin', *Am J Cardiol.*' vol. 77, pp. 545-6.

Liu, A & Stumpo, C 2007, 'Warfarin-drug interactions among older adults', *Geriatrics Aging*, vol. 10 no. 10, pp. 643-646.

Murphy, JE 2011, *Clinical pharmacokinetics*, American Society of Health-System Pharmacists, Bethesda.

Oh, DY, Talukdar, S, Bae, EJ, Imamura, T, Morinaga, H, Fan, W, Li, P, Lu, WJ, Watkins, SM & Olefsky, JM 2010. 'GPR120 is an omega-3 fatty acidreceptor mediating potent anti-inflammatory and insulin-sensitizingeffects', *Cell*, vol. 142, pp. 687–98.

Paterson, JM, Mamdani, M, Juurlink, DN, Naglie, G, Laupacis, A & Stukel, TA 2006, 'Clinical consequences of generic warfarin substitution: an ecological study', *JAMA*, vol. 296, pp. 1969-72.

Simon, E, Gariepy, J, Cogny, A, Moatti, A & Simon, A 2001, 'Erythrocyte, but not plasma, vitamin E concentration is associated with carotid intima–media thickening in asymptomatic men at risk for cardiovascular disease', *Atherosclerosis*, vol. 159, pp. 193–200.

Stenton, SB, Bungard, TJ & Ackman, M 2001, 'Interactions between Warfarin and Herbal Products, Minerals, and Vitamins: A Pharmacist's Guide', *C J H P*, vol. 54 no. 3, pp. 186-192.

1. Buckley, MS, Goff, AD & Knapp, WE 2004, 'Fish oil interaction with warfarin', *Annals of Pharmacotherapy*, vol. 38, pp. 50-53.

YOUR KNOWLEDGE HAS VALUE

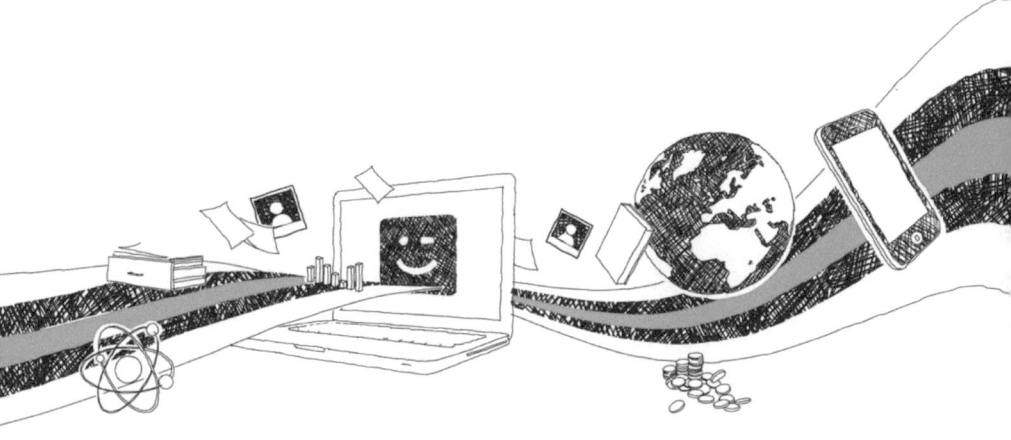

- We will publish your bachelor's and master's thesis, essays and papers

- Your own eBook and book - sold worldwide in all relevant shops

- Earn money with each sale

Upload your text at www.GRIN.com
and publish for free

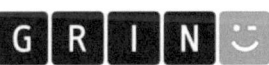